Morning

I am grateful for..

- An old relationship:

- An opportunity you have today:

- Something good/great that happened yesterday:

- Something small:

Daily affirmations I am...

Evening   Time:_____

Three amazing things that happened today...

How could I have made today better?

Morning

I am grateful for...

- An old relationship:

- An opportunity you have today:

- Something good/great that happened yesterday:

- Something small:

Daily affirmations I am...

Evening

Time:_____

Three amazing things that happened today...

How could I have made today better?

Morning

I am grateful for...

- An old relationship:

- An opportunity you have today:

- Something good/great that happened yesterday:

- Something small:

Daily affirmations I am...

Evening

Time:_____

Three amazing things that happened today...

How could I have made today better?

Morning

I am grateful for...

- An old relationship:

- An opportunity you have today:

- Something good/great that happened yesterday:

- Something small:

Daily affirmations I am...

Evening

Time:_____

Three amazing things that happened today...

How could I have made today better?

Morning

I am grateful for...

- An old relationship:

- An opportunity you have today:

- Something good/great that happened yesterday:

- Something small:

Daily affirmations I am...

Evening

Time:_____

Three amazing things that happened today...

How could I have made today better?

Morning

I am grateful for...

- An old relationship:

- An opportunity you have today:

- Something good/great that happened yesterday:

- Something small:

Daily affirmations I am...

Evening

Time:_____

Three amazing things that happened today...·

How could I have made today better?

Morning

Time:_____ Date: / /

I am grateful for...

- An old relationship:

- An opportunity you have today:

- Something good/great that happened yesterday:

- Something small:

Daily affirmations I am...

Evening

Time:_____

Three amazing things that happened today...

How could I have made today better?

Morning

I am grateful for...

- An old relationship:

- An opportunity you have today:

- Something good/great that happened yesterday:

- Something small:

Daily affirmations I am...

Evening

Time:_____

Three amazing things that happened today...

How could I have made today better?

Morning

I am grateful for...

- An old relationship:

- An opportunity you have today:

- Something good/great that happened yesterday:

- Something small:

Daily affirmations I am...

Evening

Time:_____

Three amazing things that happened today...

How could I have made today better?

Morning

I am grateful for...

- An old relationship:

- An opportunity you have today:

- Something good/great that happened yesterday:

- Something small:

Daily affirmations I am...

Evening

Time:_____

Three amazing things that happened today...

How could I have made today better?

Morning

Time:_____ Date: / /

I am grateful for...

- An old relationship:

- An opportunity you have today:

- Something good/great that happened yesterday:

- Something small:

Daily affirmations I am...

Evening

Time:_____

Three amazing things that happened today...

How could I have made today better?

Morning

Time:_____ Date: / /

I am grateful for...

- An old relationship:

- An opportunity you have today:

- Something good/great that happened yesterday:

- Something small:

Daily affirmations I am...

Evening

Time:_____

Three amazing things that happened today...

How could I have made today better?

Morning

I am grateful for...

- An old relationship:

- An opportunity you have today:

- Something good/great that happened yesterday:

- Something small:

Daily affirmations I am...

Evening

Time:_____

Three amazing things that happened today...

How could I have made today better?

Morning

I am grateful for...

- An old relationship:

- An opportunity you have today:

- Something good/great that happened yesterday:

- Something small:

Daily affirmations I am...

Evening

Time:_____

Three amazing things that happened today...

How could I have made today better?

Morning   Time:_____   Date: / /

I am grateful for...

- An old relationship:

- An opportunity you have today:

- Something good/great that happened yesterday:

- Something small:

Daily affirmations I am...

Evening   Time:_____

Three amazing things that happened today...

How could I have made today better?

Morning

I am grateful for...

- An old relationship:

- An opportunity you have today:

- Something good/great that happened yesterday:

- Something small:

Daily affirmations I am...

Evening

Time:_____

Three amazing things that happened today...

How could I have made today better?

Morning   Time:_____   Date: / /

I am grateful for...

- An old relationship:

- An opportunity you have today:

- Something good/great that happened yesterday:

- Something small:

Daily affirmations I am...

Evening   Time:_____

Three amazing things that happened today...

How could I have made today better?

Morning

I am grateful for...

- An old relationship:

- An opportunity you have today:

- Something good/great that happened yesterday:

- Something small:

Daily affirmations I am...

Evening

Time:_____

Three amazing things that happened today...

How could I have made today better?

Morning

I am grateful for...

- An old relationship:

- An opportunity you have today:

- Something good/great that happened yesterday:

- Something small:

Daily affirmations I am...

Evening

Time:_____

Three amazing things that happened today...

How could I have made today better?

Morning

I am grateful for...

- An old relationship:

- An opportunity you have today:

- Something good/great that happened yesterday:

- Something small:

Daily affirmations I am...

Evening

Time:_____

Three amazing things that happened today...

How could I have made today better?

Morning

I am grateful for...

- An old relationship:

- An opportunity you have today:

- Something good/great that happened yesterday:

- Something small:

Daily affirmations I am...

Evening

Time:_____

Three amazing things that happened today...

How could I have made today better?

Morning

Time:_____ Date: / /

I am grateful for...

- An old relationship:

- An opportunity you have today:

- Something good/great that happened yesterday:

- Something small:

Daily affirmations I am...

Evening

Time:_____

Three amazing things that happened today...

How could I have made today better?

Morning   Time:_____ Date: / /

I am grateful for...

- An old relationship:

- An opportunity you have today:

- Something good/great that happened yesterday:

- Something small:

Daily affirmations I am...

Evening   Time:_____

Three amazing things that happened today...

How could I have made today better?

Morning

Time:_____ Date: / /

I am grateful for...

- An old relationship:

- An opportunity you have today:

- Something good/great that happened yesterday:

- Something small:

Daily affirmations I am...

Evening

Time:_____

Three amazing things that happened today...

- .

How could I have made today better?

Morning

I am grateful for...

- An old relationship:

- An opportunity you have today:

- Something good/great that happened yesterday:

- Something small:

Daily affirmations I am...

Evening

Time:_____

Three amazing things that happened today...

How could I have made today better?

Morning

Time:_____ Date: / /

I am grateful for...

- An old relationship:

- An opportunity you have today:

- Something good/great that happened yesterday:

- Something small:

Daily affirmations I am...

Evening

Time:_____

Three amazing things that happened today...

How could I have made today better?

Morning

Time:_____ Date: / /

I am grateful for...

- An old relationship:

- An opportunity you have today:

- Something good/great that happened yesterday:

- Something small:

Daily affirmations I am...

Evening

Time:_____

Three amazing things that happened today...

How could I have made today better?

Morning

Time:_____ Date: / /

I am grateful for...

- An old relationship:

- An opportunity you have today:

- Something good/great that happened yesterday:

- Something small:

Daily affirmations I am...

Evening

Time:_____

Three amazing things that happened today...

How could I have made today better?

Morning

Time:_____ Date: / /

I am grateful for...

- An old relationship:

- An opportunity you have today:

- Something good/great that happened yesterday:

- Something small:

Daily affirmations I am...

Evening

Time:_____

Three amazing things that happened today...

How could I have made today better?

Morning

I am grateful for...

- An old relationship:

- An opportunity you have today:

- Something good/great that happened yesterday:

- Something small:

Daily affirmations I am...

Evening

Time:_____

Three amazing things that happened today...

How could I have made today better?

Morning

I am grateful for...

- An old relationship:

- An opportunity you have today:

- Something good/great that happened yesterday:

- Something small:

Daily affirmations I am...

Evening

Time:_____

Three amazing things that happened today...

How could I have made today better?

Morning

I am grateful for...

- An old relationship:

- An opportunity you have today:

- Something good/great that happened yesterday:

- Something small:

Daily affirmations I am...

Evening

Time:_____

Three amazing things that happened today...

How could I have made today better?

Morning

Time:_____ Date: / /

I am grateful for...

- An old relationship:

- An opportunity you have today:

- Something good/great that happened yesterday:

- Something small:

Daily affirmations I am...

Evening

Time:_____

Three amazing things that happened today...

How could I have made today better?

Morning

I am grateful for...

- An old relationship:

- An opportunity you have today:

- Something good/great that happened yesterday:

- Something small:

Daily affirmations I am...

Evening

Time:_____

Three amazing things that happened today...

How could I have made today better?

Morning

Time:_____ Date: / /

I am grateful for...

- An old relationship:

- An opportunity you have today:

- Something good/great that happened yesterday:

- Something small:

Daily affirmations I am...

Evening

Time:_____

Three amazing things that happened today...

How could I have made today better?

Morning

Time:_____ Date: / /

I am grateful for...

- An old relationship:

- An opportunity you have today:

- Something good/great that happened yesterday:

- Something small:

Daily affirmations I am...

Evening

Time:_____

Three amazing things that happened today...

How could I have made today better?

Morning

I am grateful for...

- An old relationship:

- An opportunity you have today:

- Something good/great that happened yesterday:

- Something small:

Daily affirmations I am...

Evening   Time:_____

Three amazing things that happened today...

How could I have made today better?

Morning

I am grateful for...

- An old relationship:

- An opportunity you have today:

- Something good/great that happened yesterday:

- Something small:

Daily affirmations I am...

Evening

Time:_____

Three amazing things that happened today...

How could I have made today better?

Morning

I am grateful for...

- An old relationship:

- An opportunity you have today:

- Something good/great that happened yesterday:

- Something small:

Daily affirmations I am...

Evening

Three amazing things that happened today...

How could I have made today better?

Morning

I am grateful for...

- An old relationship:

- An opportunity you have today:

- Something good/great that happened yesterday:

- Something small:

Daily affirmations I am...

Evening

Time:_____

Three amazing things that happened today...

How could I have made today better?

Morning

Time:_____ Date: / /

I am grateful for...

- An old relationship:

- An opportunity you have today:

- Something good/great that happened yesterday:

- Something small:

Daily affirmations I am...

Evening

Time:_____

Three amazing things that happened today...

How could I have made today better?

Morning

Time:_____ Date: / /

I am grateful for...

- An old relationship:

- An opportunity you have today:

- Something good/great that happened yesterday:

- Something small:

Daily affirmations I am...

Evening

Time:_____

Three amazing things that happened today...

How could I have made today better?

Morning

Time:_____ Date: / /

I am grateful for...

- An old relationship:

- An opportunity you have today:

- Something good/great that happened yesterday:

- Something small:

Daily affirmations I am...

Evening

Time:_____

Three amazing things that happened today...

How could I have made today better?

Morning

I am grateful for...

- An old relationship:

- An opportunity you have today:

- Something good/great that happened yesterday:

- Something small:

Daily affirmations I am...

Evening

Time:_____

Three amazing things that happened today...

How could I have made today better?

Morning

Time:_____ Date: / /

I am grateful for...

- An old relationship:

- An opportunity you have today:

- Something good/great that happened yesterday:

- Something small:

Daily affirmations I am...

Evening

Time:_____

Three amazing things that happened today...

How could I have made today better?

Morning

I am grateful for...

- An old relationship:

- An opportunity you have today:

- Something good/great that happened yesterday:

- Something small:

Daily affirmations I am...

Evening

Time:_____

Three amazing things that happened today...

How could I have made today better?

Morning

I am grateful for...

- An old relationship:

- An opportunity you have today:

- Something good/great that happened yesterday:

- Something small:

Daily affirmations I am...

Evening

Time:_____

Three amazing things that happened today...

How could I have made today better?

Morning

Time:_____ Date: / /

I am grateful for...

- An old relationship:

- An opportunity you have today:

- Something good/great that happened yesterday:

- Something small:

Daily affirmations I am...

Evening

Time:_____

Three amazing things that happened today...

How could I have made today better?

Morning
Time:_____ Date: / /

I am grateful for...

- An old relationship:

- An opportunity you have today:

- Something good/great that happened yesterday:

- Something small:

Daily affirmations I am...

Evening
Time:_____

Three amazing things that happened today...

How could I have made today better?

Morning

I am grateful for...

- An old relationship:

- An opportunity you have today:

- Something good/great that happened yesterday:

- Something small:

Daily affirmations I am...

Evening

Time:_____

Three amazing things that happened today...

How could I have made today better?

Morning

I am grateful for...

- An old relationship:

- An opportunity you have today:

- Something good/great that happened yesterday:

- Something small:

Daily affirmations I am...

Evening

Time:_____

Three amazing things that happened today...

How could I have made today better?

Morning

I am grateful for...

- An old relationship:

- An opportunity you have today:

- Something good/great that happened yesterday:

- Something small:

Daily affirmations I am...

Evening

Time:_____

Three amazing things that happened today...

How could I have made today better?

Morning

Time:_____   Date: /   /

I am grateful for...

- An old relationship:

- An opportunity you have today:

- Something good/great that happened yesterday:

- Something small:

Daily affirmations I am...

Evening

Time:_____

Three amazing things that happened today...

How could I have made today better?

Morning

I am grateful for...

- An old relationship:

- An opportunity you have today:

- Something good/great that happened yesterday:

- Something small:

Daily affirmations I am...

Evening

Time:_____

Three amazing things that happened today...

How could I have made today better?

Morning

Time:_____ Date: / /

I am grateful for...

- An old relationship:

- An opportunity you have today:

- Something good/great that happened yesterday:

- Something small:

Daily affirmations I am...

Evening

Time:_____

Three amazing things that happened today...

How could I have made today better?

Morning

I am grateful for...

- An old relationship:

- An opportunity you have today:

- Something good/great that happened yesterday:

- Something small:

Daily affirmations I am...

Evening

Time:_____

Three amazing things that happened today...

How could I have made today better?

Morning

Time:_____ Date: / /

I am grateful for...

- An old relationship:

- An opportunity you have today:

- Something good/great that happened yesterday:

- Something small:

Daily affirmations I am...

Evening

Time:_____

Three amazing things that happened today...

How could I have made today better?

Morning

Time:_____ Date: / /

I am grateful for...

- An old relationship:

- An opportunity you have today:

- Something good/great that happened yesterday:

- Something small:

Daily affirmations I am...

Evening

Time:_____

Three amazing things that happened today...

How could I have made today better?

Morning

I am grateful for...

- An old relationship:

- An opportunity you have today:

- Something good/great that happened yesterday:

- Something small:

Daily affirmations I am...

Evening

Time:_____

Three amazing things that happened today...

How could I have made today better?

Morning

I am grateful for...

- An old relationship:

- An opportunity you have today:

- Something good/great that happened yesterday:

- Something small:

Daily affirmations I am...

Evening

Time:_____

Three amazing things that happened today...

How could I have made today better?

Morning

I am grateful for...

- An old relationship:

- An opportunity you have today:

- Something good/great that happened yesterday:

- Something small:

Daily affirmations I am...

Evening

Time:_____

Three amazing things that happened today...

How could I have made today better?

Morning

I am grateful for...

- An old relationship:

- An opportunity you have today:

- Something good/great that happened yesterday:

- Something small:

Daily affirmations I am...

Evening

Time:_____

Three amazing things that happened today...

How could I have made today better?

Morning

I am grateful for...

- An old relationship:

- An opportunity you have today:

- Something good/great that happened yesterday:

- Something small:

Daily affirmations I am...

Evening
Time:_____

Three amazing things that happened today...

How could I have made today better?

Morning

Time:_____ Date: / /

I am grateful for...

- An old relationship:

- An opportunity you have today:

- Something good/great that happened yesterday:

- Something small:

Daily affirmations I am...

Evening

Time:_____

Three amazing things that happened today...

How could I have made today better?

Morning

Time:_____ Date: / /

I am grateful for...

- An old relationship:

- An opportunity you have today:

- Something good/great that happened yesterday:

- Something small:

Daily affirmations I am...

Evening

Time:_____

Three amazing things that happened today...

How could I have made today better?

Morning

Time:_____ Date: / /

I am grateful for...

- An old relationship:

- An opportunity you have today:

- Something good/great that happened yesterday:

- Something small:

Daily affirmations I am...

Evening

Time:_____

Three amazing things that happened today...

How could I have made today better?

Morning

Time:_____ Date: / /

I am grateful for...

- An old relationship:

- An opportunity you have today:

- Something good/great that happened yesterday:

- Something small:

Daily affirmations I am...

Evening

Time:_____

Three amazing things that happened today...

How could I have made today better?

Morning

Time:_____ Date: / /

I am grateful for...

- An old relationship:

- An opportunity you have today:

- Something good/great that happened yesterday:

- Something small:

Daily affirmations I am...

Evening

Time:_____

Three amazing things that happened today...

How could I have made today better?

Morning

I am grateful for...

- An old relationship:

- An opportunity you have today:

- Something good/great that happened yesterday:

- Something small:

Daily affirmations I am...

Evening

Time:_____

Three amazing things that happened today...

How could I have made today better?

Morning

I am grateful for...

- An old relationship:

- An opportunity you have today:

- Something good/great that happened yesterday:

- Something small:

Daily affirmations I am...

Evening

Time:_____

Three amazing things that happened today...

How could I have made today better?

Morning

I am grateful for...

- An old relationship:

- An opportunity you have today:

- Something good/great that happened yesterday:

- Something small:

Daily affirmations I am...

Evening

Time:_____

Three amazing things that happened today...

How could I have made today better?

Morning

Time:_____ Date: / /

I am grateful for...

- An old relationship:

- An opportunity you have today:

- Something good/great that happened yesterday:

- Something small:

Daily affirmations I am...

Evening

Time:_____

Three amazing things that happened today...

How could I have made today better?

Morning

I am grateful for...

- An old relationship:

- An opportunity you have today:

- Something good/great that happened yesterday:

- Something small:

Daily affirmations I am...

Evening

Time:_____

Three amazing things that happened today...

How could I have made today better?

Morning

I am grateful for...

- An old relationship:

- An opportunity you have today:

- Something good/great that happened yesterday:

- Something small:

Daily affirmations I am...

Evening

Time:_____

Three amazing things that happened today...

How could I have made today better?

Morning

I am grateful for...

- An old relationship:

- An opportunity you have today:

- Something good/great that happened yesterday:

- Something small:

Daily affirmations I am...

Evening

Time:_____

Three amazing things that happened today...

How could I have made today better?

Morning

I am grateful for...

- An old relationship:

- An opportunity you have today:

- Something good/great that happened yesterday:

- Something small:

Daily affirmations I am...

Evening

Time:_____

Three amazing things that happened today...

How could I have made today better?

Morning

Time:_____ Date: / /

I am grateful for...

- An old relationship:

- An opportunity you have today:

- Something good/great that happened yesterday:

- Something small:

Daily affirmations I am...

Evening

Time:_____

Three amazing things that happened today...

How could I have made today better?

Morning

I am grateful for...

- An old relationship:

- An opportunity you have today:

- Something good/great that happened yesterday:

- Something small:

Daily affirmations I am...

Evening

Time:_____

Three amazing things that happened today...

How could I have made today better?

Morning

I am grateful for...

- • An old relationship:

- • An opportunity you have today:

- • Something good/great that happened yesterday:

- • Something small:

Daily affirmations I am...

Evening

Time:_____

Three amazing things that happened today...

How could I have made today better?

Morning

I am grateful for...

- An old relationship:

- An opportunity you have today:

- Something good/great that happened yesterday:

- Something small:

Daily affirmations I am...

Evening

Time:_____

Three amazing things that happened today...

How could I have made today better?

Morning

I am grateful for...

- An old relationship:

- An opportunity you have today:

- Something good/great that happened yesterday:

- Something small:

Daily affirmations I am...

Evening

Time:_____

Three amazing things that happened today...

How could I have made today better?

Morning

Time:_____ Date: / /

I am grateful for...

- An old relationship:

- An opportunity you have today:

- Something good/great that happened yesterday:

- Something small:

Daily affirmations I am...

Evening

Time:_____

Three amazing things that happened today...

How could I have made today better?

Morning

Time:_____ Date: / /

I am grateful for...

- An old relationship:

- An opportunity you have today:

- Something good/great that happened yesterday:

- Something small:

Daily affirmations I am...

Evening

Time:_____

Three amazing things that happened today...

How could I have made today better?

Morning

I am grateful for...

- An old relationship:

- An opportunity you have today:

- Something good/great that happened yesterday:

- Something small:

Daily affirmations I am...

Evening

Time:_____

Three amazing things that happened today...

How could I have made today better?

Morning

I am grateful for...

- An old relationship:

- An opportunity you have today:

- Something good/great that happened yesterday:

- Something small:

Daily affirmations I am...

Evening

Time:_____

Three amazing things that happened today...

How could I have made today better?

Morning

I am grateful for...

- An old relationship:

- An opportunity you have today:

- Something good/great that happened yesterday:

- Something small:

Daily affirmations I am...

Evening

Time:_____

Three amazing things that happened today...

How could I have made today better?

Morning

I am grateful for...

- An old relationship:

- An opportunity you have today:

- Something good/great that happened yesterday:

- Something small:

Daily affirmations I am...

Evening

Time:_____

Three amazing things that happened today...

How could I have made today better?

Morning

I am grateful for...

- An old relationship:

- An opportunity you have today:

- Something good/great that happened yesterday:

- Something small:

Daily affirmations I am...

Evening

Time:_____

Three amazing things that happened today...

How could I have made today better?

Morning

Time:_____ Date: / /

I am grateful for...

- An old relationship:

- An opportunity you have today:

- Something good/great that happened yesterday:

- Something small:

Daily affirmations I am...

Evening

Time:_____

Three amazing things that happened today...

How could I have made today better?

Morning

Time:_____ Date: / /

I am grateful for...

- An old relationship:

- An opportunity you have today:

- Something good/great that happened yesterday:

- Something small:

Daily affirmations I am...

Evening

Time:_____

Three amazing things that happened today...

How could I have made today better?

Morning

Time:_____ Date: / /

I am grateful for...

- An old relationship:

- An opportunity you have today:

- Something good/great that happened yesterday:

- Something small:

Daily affirmations I am...

Evening

Time:_____

Three amazing things that happened today...

How could I have made today better?

Morning

I am grateful for...

- An old relationship:

- An opportunity you have today:

- Something good/great that happened yesterday:

- Something small:

Daily affirmations I am...

Evening

Time:_____

Three amazing things that happened today...

How could I have made today better?

Morning

I am grateful for...

- An old relationship:

- An opportunity you have today:

- Something good/great that happened yesterday:

- Something small:

Daily affirmations I am...

Evening

Time:_____

Three amazing things that happened today...

How could I have made today better?

Morning

Time:_____   Date: / /

I am grateful for...

- An old relationship:

- An opportunity you have today:

- Something good/great that happened yesterday:

- Something small:

Daily affirmations I am...

Evening

Time:_____

Three amazing things that happened today...

How could I have made today better?

Morning

Time:_____ Date: / /

I am grateful for...

- An old relationship:

- An opportunity you have today:

- Something good/great that happened yesterday:

- Something small:

Daily affirmations I am...

Evening

Time:_____

Three amazing things that happened today...

How could I have made today better?

Morning

I am grateful for...

- An old relationship:

- An opportunity you have today:

- Something good/great that happened yesterday:

- Something small:

Daily affirmations I am...

Evening

Time:_____

Three amazing things that happened today...

How could I have made today better?

Morning

I am grateful for...

- An old relationship:

- An opportunity you have today:

- Something good/great that happened yesterday:

- Something small:

Daily affirmations I am...

Evening

Time:_____

Three amazing things that happened today...

How could I have made today better?

Morning

I am grateful for...

- An old relationship:

- An opportunity you have today:

- Something good/great that happened yesterday:

- Something small:

Daily affirmations I am...

Evening

Time:_____

Three amazing things that happened today...

How could I have made today better?

Morning

Time:_____ Date: / /

I am grateful for...

- An old relationship:

- An opportunity you have today:

- Something good/great that happened yesterday:

- Something small:

Daily affirmations I am...

Evening

Time:_____

Three amazing things that happened today...

How could I have made today better?

Morning

Time:_____ Date: / /

I am grateful for...

- An old relationship:

- An opportunity you have today:

- Something good/great that happened yesterday:

- Something small:

Daily affirmations I am...

Evening

Time:_____

Three amazing things that happened today...

How could I have made today better?

Morning Time:_____ Date: / /

I am grateful for...

- An old relationship:

- An opportunity you have today:

- Something good/great that happened yesterday:

- Something small:

Daily affirmations I am...

Evening Time:_____

Three amazing things that happened today...

How could I have made today better?

Morning

I am grateful for...

- An old relationship:

- An opportunity you have today:

- Something good/great that happened yesterday:

- Something small:

Daily affirmations I am...

Evening

Time:_____

Three amazing things that happened today...

How could I have made today better?

Morning

I am grateful for...

- An old relationship:

- An opportunity you have today:

- Something good/great that happened yesterday:

- Something small:

Daily affirmations I am...

Evening

Three amazing things that happened today...

How could I have made today better?

Morning

I am grateful for...

- An old relationship:

- An opportunity you have today:

- Something good/great that happened yesterday:

- Something small:

Daily affirmations I am...

Evening

Time:_____

Three amazing things that happened today...

How could I have made today better?

Morning   Time:_____ Date: / /

I am grateful for...

- An old relationship:

- An opportunity you have today:

- Something good/great that happened yesterday:

- Something small:

Daily affirmations I am...

Evening   Time:_____

Three amazing things that happened today...

How could I have made today better?

Morning

Time:_____ Date: / /

I am grateful for...

- An old relationship:

- An opportunity you have today:

- Something good/great that happened yesterday:

- Something small:

Daily affirmations I am...

Evening

Time:_____

Three amazing things that happened today...

How could I have made today better?

Morning

I am grateful for...

- An old relationship:

- An opportunity you have today:

- Something good/great that happened yesterday:

- Something small:

Daily affirmations I am...

Evening

Time:_____

Three amazing things that happened today...

How could I have made today better?

Morning

I am grateful for...

- An old relationship:

- An opportunity you have today:

- Something good/great that happened yesterday:

- Something small:

Daily affirmations I am...

Evening

Time:_____

Three amazing things that happened today...

How could I have made today better?

Morning

I am grateful for...

- An old relationship:

- An opportunity you have today:

- Something good/great that happened yesterday:

- Something small:

Daily affirmations I am...

Evening

Time:_____

Three amazing things that happened today...

How could I have made today better?

Morning

Time:_____ Date: / /

I am grateful for...

- An old relationship:

- An opportunity you have today:

- Something good/great that happened yesterday:

- Something small:

Daily affirmations I am...

Evening

Time:_____

Three amazing things that happened today...

How could I have made today better?

Morning

I am grateful for...

- An old relationship:

- An opportunity you have today:

- Something good/great that happened yesterday:

- Something small:

Daily affirmations I am...

Evening

Time:_____

Three amazing things that happened today...

How could I have made today better?

Morning

I am grateful for...

- An old relationship:

- An opportunity you have today:

- Something good/great that happened yesterday:

- Something small:

Daily affirmations I am...

Evening

Time:_____

Three amazing things that happened today...

How could I have made today better?

Morning

Time:_____ Date: / /

I am grateful for...

- An old relationship:

- An opportunity you have today:

- Something good/great that happened yesterday:

- Something small:

Daily affirmations I am...

Evening

Time:_____

Three amazing things that happened today...

How could I have made today better?

Morning

Time:_____ Date: / /

I am grateful for...

- An old relationship:

- An opportunity you have today:

- Something good/great that happened yesterday:

- Something small:

Daily affirmations I am...

Evening

Time:_____

Three amazing things that happened today...

How could I have made today better?

Morning   Time:_____ Date: / /

I am grateful for...

- An old relationship:

- An opportunity you have today:

- Something good/great that happened yesterday:

- Something small:

Daily affirmations I am...

Evening   Time:_____

Three amazing things that happened today...

How could I have made today better?

Morning

I am grateful for...

- An old relationship:

- An opportunity you have today:

- Something good/great that happened yesterday:

- Something small:

Daily affirmations I am...

Evening

Time:_____

Three amazing things that happened today...

How could I have made today better?

Morning

I am grateful for...

- An old relationship:

- An opportunity you have today:

- Something good/great that happened yesterday:

- Something small:

Daily affirmations I am...

Evening

Time:_____

Three amazing things that happened today...

How could I have made today better?

Morning

I am grateful for...

- An old relationship:

- An opportunity you have today:

- Something good/great that happened yesterday:

- Something small:

Daily affirmations I am...

Evening

Time:_____

Three amazing things that happened today...

How could I have made today better?

Morning

I am grateful for...

- An old relationship:

- An opportunity you have today:

- Something good/great that happened yesterday:

- Something small:

Daily affirmations I am...

Evening

Time:_____

Three amazing things that happened today...

How could I have made today better?

Morning

I am grateful for...

- An old relationship:

- An opportunity you have today:

- Something good/great that happened yesterday:

- Something small:

Daily affirmations I am...

Evening

Time:_____

Three amazing things that happened today...

How could I have made today better?

Morning

I am grateful for...

- An old relationship:

- An opportunity you have today:

- Something good/great that happened yesterday:

- Something small:

Daily affirmations I am...

Evening

Time:_____

Three amazing things that happened today...

How could I have made today better?

Morning

I am grateful for...

- An old relationship:

- An opportunity you have today:

- Something good/great that happened yesterday:

- Something small:

Daily affirmations I am...

Evening

Time:_____

Three amazing things that happened today...

How could I have made today better?

Morning

Time:_____ Date: / /

I am grateful for...

- An old relationship:

- An opportunity you have today:

- Something good/great that happened yesterday:

- Something small:

Daily affirmations I am...

Evening

Time:_____

Three amazing things that happened today...

How could I have made today better?

Morning

I am grateful for...

- An old relationship:

- An opportunity you have today:

- Something good/great that happened yesterday:

- Something small:

Daily affirmations I am...

Evening

Time:_____

Three amazing things that happened today...

How could I have made today better?

Morning

I am grateful for...

- An old relationship:

- An opportunity you have today:

- Something good/great that happened yesterday:

- Something small:

Daily affirmations I am...

Evening

Time:_____

Three amazing things that happened today...

How could I have made today better?

Morning

I am grateful for...

- • An old relationship:

- • An opportunity you have today:

- • Something good/great that happened yesterday:

- • Something small:

Daily affirmations I am...

Evening

Time:_____

Three amazing things that happened today...

How could I have made today better?

Morning   Time:_____   Date: / /

I am grateful for...

- An old relationship:

- An opportunity you have today:

- Something good/great that happened yesterday:

- Something small:

Daily affirmations I am...

Evening   Time:_____

Three amazing things that happened today...

How could I have made today better?

Morning

Time:_____ Date: / /

I am grateful for...

- An old relationship:

- An opportunity you have today:

- Something good/great that happened yesterday:

- Something small:

Daily affirmations I am...

Evening

Time:_____

Three amazing things that happened today...

How could I have made today better?

Morning

I am grateful for...

- • An old relationship:

- • An opportunity you have today:

- • Something good/great that happened yesterday:

- • Something small:

Daily affirmations I am...

Evening

Time:_____

Three amazing things that happened today...

How could I have made today better?

Morning

I am grateful for...

- An old relationship:

- An opportunity you have today:

- Something good/great that happened yesterday:

- Something small:

Daily affirmations I am...

Evening

Time:_____

Three amazing things that happened today...

How could I have made today better?

Morning

Time:_____   Date: / /

I am grateful for...

- An old relationship:

- An opportunity you have today:

- Something good/great that happened yesterday:

- Something small:

Daily affirmations I am...

Evening

Time:_____

Three amazing things that happened today...

How could I have made today better?

Morning

Time:_____ Date: / /

I am grateful for...

- An old relationship:

- An opportunity you have today:

- Something good/great that happened yesterday:

- Something small:

Daily affirmations I am...

Evening

Time:_____

Three amazing things that happened today...

How could I have made today better?

Morning

I am grateful for...

- An old relationship:

- An opportunity you have today:

- Something good/great that happened yesterday:

- Something small:

Daily affirmations I am...

Evening

Time:_____

Three amazing things that happened today...

How could I have made today better?

Morning

I am grateful for...

- An old relationship:

- An opportunity you have today:

- Something good/great that happened yesterday:

- Something small:

Daily affirmations I am...

Evening

Time:_____

Three amazing things that happened today...

How could I have made today better?

Morning

Time:_____ Date: / /

I am grateful for...

- An old relationship:

- An opportunity you have today:

- Something good/great that happened yesterday:

- Something small:

Daily affirmations I am...

Evening

Time:_____

Three amazing things that happened today...

How could I have made today better?

Morning

Time:_____ Date: / /

I am grateful for...

- An old relationship:

- An opportunity you have today:

- Something good/great that happened yesterday:

- Something small:

Daily affirmations I am...

Evening

Time:_____

Three amazing things that happened today...

How could I have made today better?

Morning

I am grateful for...

- An old relationship:

- An opportunity you have today:

- Something good/great that happened yesterday:

- Something small:

Daily affirmations I am...

Evening

Time:_____

Three amazing things that happened today...

How could I have made today better?

Morning

I am grateful for...

- An old relationship:

- An opportunity you have today:

- Something good/great that happened yesterday:

- Something small:

Daily affirmations I am...

Evening

Time:_____

Three amazing things that happened today...

How could I have made today better?

Morning

I am grateful for…

- An old relationship:

- An opportunity you have today:

- Something good/great that happened yesterday:

- Something small:

Daily affirmations I am...

Evening

Time:_____

Three amazing things that happened today…

How could I have made today better?

Morning

Time:_____ Date: / /

I am grateful for...

- An old relationship:

- An opportunity you have today:

- Something good/great that happened yesterday:

- Something small:

Daily affirmations I am...

Evening

Time:_____

Three amazing things that happened today...

How could I have made today better?

Morning

Time:_____ Date: / /

I am grateful for...

- An old relationship:

- An opportunity you have today:

- Something good/great that happened yesterday:

- Something small:

Daily affirmations I am...

Evening

Time:_____

Three amazing things that happened today...

How could I have made today better?

Morning

I am grateful for...

- An old relationship:

- An opportunity you have today:

- Something good/great that happened yesterday:

- Something small:

Daily affirmations I am...

Evening

Time:_____

Three amazing things that happened today...

How could I have made today better?

Morning

I am grateful for...

- An old relationship:

- An opportunity you have today:

- Something good/great that happened yesterday:

- Something small:

Daily affirmations I am...

Evening

Time:_____

Three amazing things that happened today...

How could I have made today better?

Morning

I am grateful for...

- An old relationship:

- An opportunity you have today:

- Something good/great that happened yesterday:

- Something small:

Daily affirmations I am...

Evening

Time:_____

Three amazing things that happened today...

How could I have made today better?

Morning

I am grateful for...

- • An old relationship:

- • An opportunity you have today:

- • Something good/great that happened yesterday:

- • Something small:

Daily affirmations I am...

Evening

Three amazing things that happened today...

How could I have made today better?

Morning

Time:_____ Date: / /

I am grateful for...

- An old relationship:

- An opportunity you have today:

- Something good/great that happened yesterday:

- Something small:

Daily affirmations I am...

Evening

Time:_____

Three amazing things that happened today...

How could I have made today better?

Morning

Time:_____ Date: / /

I am grateful for...

- An old relationship:

- An opportunity you have today:

- Something good/great that happened yesterday:

- Something small:

Daily affirmations I am...

Evening

Time:_____

Three amazing things that happened today...

How could I have made today better?

Morning

I am grateful for...

- An old relationship:

- An opportunity you have today:

- Something good/great that happened yesterday:

- Something small:

Daily affirmations I am...

Evening

Time:_____

Three amazing things that happened today...

How could I have made today better?

Morning

I am grateful for...

- An old relationship:

- An opportunity you have today:

- Something good/great that happened yesterday:

- Something small:

Daily affirmations I am...

Evening

Time:_____

Three amazing things that happened today...

How could I have made today better?

Morning

I am grateful for...

- An old relationship:

- An opportunity you have today:

- Something good/great that happened yesterday:

- Something small:

Daily affirmations I am...

Evening

Time:_____

Three amazing things that happened today...

How could I have made today better?

Morning

I am grateful for...

- An old relationship:

- An opportunity you have today:

- Something good/great that happened yesterday:

- Something small:

Daily affirmations I am...

Evening

Time:_____

Three amazing things that happened today...

How could I have made today better?

Morning

I am grateful for...

- An old relationship:

- An opportunity you have today:

- Something good/great that happened yesterday:

- Something small:

Daily affirmations I am...

Evening

Time:_____

Three amazing things that happened today...

How could I have made today better?

Morning

Time:_____ Date: / /

I am grateful for...

- An old relationship:

- An opportunity you have today:

- Something good/great that happened yesterday:

- Something small:

Daily affirmations I am...

Evening

Time:_____

Three amazing things that happened today...

How could I have made today better?

Morning

I am grateful for...

- An old relationship:

- An opportunity you have today:

- Something good/great that happened yesterday:

- Something small:

Daily affirmations I am...

Evening

Time:_____

Three amazing things that happened today...

How could I have made today better?

Morning

I am grateful for...

- An old relationship:

- An opportunity you have today:

- Something good/great that happened yesterday:

- Something small:

Daily affirmations I am...

Evening

Time:_____

Three amazing things that happened today...

How could I have made today better?

Morning

I am grateful for...

- An old relationship:

- An opportunity you have today:

- Something good/great that happened yesterday:

- Something small:

Daily affirmations I am...

Evening

Time:_____

Three amazing things that happened today...

How could I have made today better?

Morning

Time:_____ Date: / /

I am grateful for...

- An old relationship:

- An opportunity you have today:

- Something good/great that happened yesterday:

- Something small:

Daily affirmations I am...

Evening

Time:_____

Three amazing things that happened today...

How could I have made today better?

Morning

I am grateful for...

- An old relationship:

- An opportunity you have today:

- Something good/great that happened yesterday:

- Something small:

Daily affirmations I am...

Evening

Time:_____

Three amazing things that happened today...

How could I have made today better?

Morning

Time:_____ Date: / /

I am grateful for...

- An old relationship:

- An opportunity you have today:

- Something good/great that happened yesterday:

- Something small:

Daily affirmations I am...

Evening

Time:_____

Three amazing things that happened today...

How could I have made today better?

Morning

I am grateful for...

- An old relationship:

- An opportunity you have today:

- Something good/great that happened yesterday:

- Something small:

Daily affirmations I am...

Evening

Time:_____

Three amazing things that happened today...

How could I have made today better?

Morning

Time:_____ Date: / /

I am grateful for...

- An old relationship:

- An opportunity you have today:

- Something good/great that happened yesterday:

- Something small:

Daily affirmations I am...

Evening

Time:_____

Three amazing things that happened today...

How could I have made today better?

Morning

I am grateful for...

- An old relationship:

- An opportunity you have today:

- Something good/great that happened yesterday:

- Something small:

Daily affirmations I am...

Evening

Time:_____

Three amazing things that happened today...

How could I have made today better?

Morning

I am grateful for...

- An old relationship:

- An opportunity you have today:

- Something good/great that happened yesterday:

- Something small:

Daily affirmations I am...

Evening

Time:_____

Three amazing things that happened today...

How could I have made today better?

Morning

I am grateful for...

- An old relationship:

- An opportunity you have today:

- Something good/great that happened yesterday:

- Something small:

Daily affirmations I am...

Evening

Time:_____

Three amazing things that happened today...

How could I have made today better?

Morning

I am grateful for...

- An old relationship:

- An opportunity you have today:

- Something good/great that happened yesterday:

- Something small:

Daily affirmations I am...

Evening   Time:_____

Three amazing things that happened today...

How could I have made today better?

Morning

Time:_____ Date: / /

I am grateful for...

- An old relationship:

- An opportunity you have today:

- Something good/great that happened yesterday:

- Something small:

Daily affirmations I am...

Evening

Time:_____

Three amazing things that happened today...

How could I have made today better?

Morning

Time:_____ Date: / /

I am grateful for...

- An old relationship:

- An opportunity you have today:

- Something good/great that happened yesterday:

- Something small:

Daily affirmations I am...

Evening

Time:_____

Three amazing things that happened today...

How could I have made today better?

Morning

I am grateful for...

- An old relationship:

- An opportunity you have today:

- Something good/great that happened yesterday:

- Something small:

Daily affirmations I am...

Evening

Time:_____

Three amazing things that happened today...

How could I have made today better?

Morning

I am grateful for...

- An old relationship:

- An opportunity you have today:

- Something good/great that happened yesterday:

- Something small:

Daily affirmations I am...

Evening

Time:_____

Three amazing things that happened today...

How could I have made today better?

Morning

I am grateful for...

- An old relationship:

- An opportunity you have today:

- Something good/great that happened yesterday:

- Something small:

Daily affirmations I am...

Evening

Three amazing things that happened today...

How could I have made today better?

Morning   Time:_____ Date: / /

I am grateful for...

- An old relationship:

- An opportunity you have today:

- Something good/great that happened yesterday:

- Something small:

Daily affirmations I am...

Evening   Time:_____

Three amazing things that happened today...

How could I have made today better?

Morning

Time:_____ Date: / /

I am grateful for...

- An old relationship:

- An opportunity you have today:

- Something good/great that happened yesterday:

- Something small:

Daily affirmations I am...

Evening

Time:_____

Three amazing things that happened today...

How could I have made today better?

Morning   Time:_____ Date: / /

I am grateful for...

- An old relationship:

- An opportunity you have today:

- Something good/great that happened yesterday:

- Something small:

Daily affirmations I am...

Evening   Time:_____

Three amazing things that happened today...

How could I have made today better?

Morning

Time:_____ Date: / /

I am grateful for...

- An old relationship:

- An opportunity you have today:

- Something good/great that happened yesterday:

- Something small:

Daily affirmations I am...

Evening

Time:_____

Three amazing things that happened today...

How could I have made today better?

Morning

I am grateful for...

- An old relationship:

- An opportunity you have today:

- Something good/great that happened yesterday:

- Something small:

Daily affirmations I am...

Evening

Time:_____

Three amazing things that happened today...

How could I have made today better?

Morning

I am grateful for...

- An old relationship:

- An opportunity you have today:

- Something good/great that happened yesterday:

- Something small:

Daily affirmations I am...

Evening Time:_____

Three amazing things that happened today...

How could I have made today better?

Morning

I am grateful for...

- An old relationship:

- An opportunity you have today:

- Something good/great that happened yesterday:

- Something small:

Daily affirmations I am...

Evening

Time:_____

Three amazing things that happened today...

How could I have made today better?

Morning

I am grateful for...

- An old relationship:

- An opportunity you have today:

- Something good/great that happened yesterday:

- Something small:

Daily affirmations I am...

Evening

Time:_____

Three amazing things that happened today...

How could I have made today better?

Morning

Time:_____ Date: / /

I am grateful for...

- An old relationship:

- An opportunity you have today:

- Something good/great that happened yesterday:

- Something small:

Daily affirmations I am...

Evening

Time:_____

Three amazing things that happened today...

How could I have made today better?

Morning

Time:_____ Date: / /

I am grateful for...

- An old relationship:

- An opportunity you have today:

- Something good/great that happened yesterday:

- Something small:

Daily affirmations I am...

Evening

Time:_____

Three amazing things that happened today...

How could I have made today better?

Morning

I am grateful for...

- An old relationship:

- An opportunity you have today:

- Something good/great that happened yesterday:

- Something small:

Daily affirmations I am...

Evening

Time:_____

Three amazing things that happened today...

How could I have made today better?

Morning

I am grateful for...

- An old relationship:

- An opportunity you have today:

- Something good/great that happened yesterday:

- Something small:

Daily affirmations I am...

Evening

Time:_____

Three amazing things that happened today...

How could I have made today better?

Morning

I am grateful for...

- An old relationship:

- An opportunity you have today:

- Something good/great that happened yesterday:

- Something small:

Daily affirmations I am...

Evening

Three amazing things that happened today...

How could I have made today better?

Morning

Time:_____ Date: / /

I am grateful for...

- An old relationship:

- An opportunity you have today:

- Something good/great that happened yesterday:

- Something small:

Daily affirmations I am...

Evening

Time:_____

Three amazing things that happened today...

How could I have made today better?

Morning

I am grateful for...

- An old relationship:

- An opportunity you have today:

- Something good/great that happened yesterday:

- Something small:

Daily affirmations I am...

Evening

Time:_____

Three amazing things that happened today...

How could I have made today better?

Morning

Time:_____   Date: / /

I am grateful for...

- An old relationship:

- An opportunity you have today:

- Something good/great that happened yesterday:

- Something small:

Daily affirmations I am...

Evening

Time:_____

Three amazing things that happened today...

How could I have made today better?

Morning

Time:_____ Date: / /

I am grateful for...

- An old relationship:

- An opportunity you have today:

- Something good/great that happened yesterday:

- Something small:

Daily affirmations I am...

Evening

Time:_____

Three amazing things that happened today...

How could I have made today better?

Morning

I am grateful for...

- An old relationship:

- An opportunity you have today:

- Something good/great that happened yesterday:

- Something small:

Daily affirmations I am...

Evening

Time:_____

Three amazing things that happened today...

How could I have made today better?

Morning

I am grateful for...

- An old relationship:

- An opportunity you have today:

- Something good/great that happened yesterday:

- Something small:

Daily affirmations I am...

Evening

Three amazing things that happened today...

How could I have made today better?

Morning

I am grateful for...

- An old relationship:

- An opportunity you have today:

- Something good/great that happened yesterday:

- Something small:

Daily affirmations I am...

Evening

Time:_____

Three amazing things that happened today...

How could I have made today better?

Morning

Time:_____ Date: / /

I am grateful for...

- An old relationship:

- An opportunity you have today:

- Something good/great that happened yesterday:

- Something small:

Daily affirmations I am...

Evening

Time:_____

Three amazing things that happened today...

How could I have made today better?

Morning

I am grateful for...

- An old relationship:

- An opportunity you have today:

- Something good/great that happened yesterday:

- Something small:

Daily affirmations I am...

Evening

Time:_____

Three amazing things that happened today...

How could I have made today better?

Morning

Time:_____ Date: / /

I am grateful for...

- An old relationship:

- An opportunity you have today:

- Something good/great that happened yesterday:

- Something small:

Daily affirmations I am...

Evening

Time:_____

Three amazing things that happened today...

How could I have made today better?

Morning

Time:_____ Date: / /

I am grateful for...

- An old relationship:

- An opportunity you have today:

- Something good/great that happened yesterday:

- Something small:

Daily affirmations I am...

Evening

Time:_____

Three amazing things that happened today...

How could I have made today better?

Morning

I am grateful for...

- An old relationship:

- An opportunity you have today:

- Something good/great that happened yesterday:

- Something small:

Daily affirmations I am...

Evening

Time:_____

Three amazing things that happened today...

How could I have made today better?

Morning

I am grateful for...

- An old relationship:

- An opportunity you have today:

- Something good/great that happened yesterday:

- Something small:

Daily affirmations I am...

Evening

Time:_____

Three amazing things that happened today...

How could I have made today better?

Morning

Time:_____ Date: / /

I am grateful for...

- An old relationship:

- An opportunity you have today:

- Something good/great that happened yesterday:

- Something small:

Daily affirmations I am...

Evening

Time:_____

Three amazing things that happened today...

How could I have made today better?

Morning

Time:_____ Date: / /

I am grateful for...

- An old relationship:

- An opportunity you have today:

- Something good/great that happened yesterday:

- Something small:

Daily affirmations I am...

Evening

Time:_____

Three amazing things that happened today...

How could I have made today better?

Morning   Time:_____ Date: / /

I am grateful for...

- An old relationship:

- An opportunity you have today:

- Something good/great that happened yesterday:

- Something small:

Daily affirmations I am...

Evening   Time:_____

Three amazing things that happened today...

How could I have made today better?

Morning

I am grateful for...

- An old relationship:

- An opportunity you have today:

- Something good/great that happened yesterday:

- Something small:

Daily affirmations I am...

Evening

Time:_____

Three amazing things that happened today...

How could I have made today better?

Morning

I am grateful for...

- An old relationship:

- An opportunity you have today:

- Something good/great that happened yesterday:

- Something small:

Daily affirmations I am...

Evening

Time:_____

Three amazing things that happened today...

.

How could I have made today better?

Morning

I am grateful for...

- An old relationship:

- An opportunity you have today:

- Something good/great that happened yesterday:

- Something small:

Daily affirmations I am...

Evening

Time:_____

Three amazing things that happened today...

How could I have made today better?

Morning   Time:_____ Date: / /

I am grateful for...

- An old relationship:

- An opportunity you have today:

- Something good/great that happened yesterday:

- Something small:

Daily affirmations I am...

Evening   Time:_____

Three amazing things that happened today...

How could I have made today better?

Morning

I am grateful for...

- An old relationship:

- An opportunity you have today:

- Something good/great that happened yesterday:

- Something small:

Daily affirmations I am...

Evening

Time:_____

Three amazing things that happened today...

How could I have made today better?

Morning

Time:_____ Date: / /

I am grateful for...

- An old relationship:

- An opportunity you have today:

- Something good/great that happened yesterday:

- Something small:

Daily affirmations I am...

Evening

Time:_____

Three amazing things that happened today...

How could I have made today better?

Morning

I am grateful for...

- An old relationship:

- An opportunity you have today:

- Something good/great that happened yesterday:

- Something small:

Daily affirmations I am...

Evening

Time:_____

Three amazing things that happened today...

How could I have made today better?

Morning

Time:_____ Date: / /

I am grateful for...

- An old relationship:

- An opportunity you have today:

- Something good/great that happened yesterday:

- Something small:

Daily affirmations I am...

Evening

Time:_____

Three amazing things that happened today...

How could I have made today better?

Morning

I am grateful for...

- An old relationship:

- An opportunity you have today:

- Something good/great that happened yesterday:

- Something small:

Daily affirmations I am...

Evening

Time:_____

Three amazing things that happened today...

How could I have made today better?

Morning

I am grateful for...

- An old relationship:

- An opportunity you have today:

- Something good/great that happened yesterday:

- Something small:

Daily affirmations I am...

Evening

Time:_____

Three amazing things that happened today...

How could I have made today better?

Morning

I am grateful for...

- An old relationship:

- An opportunity you have today:

- Something good/great that happened yesterday:

- Something small:

Daily affirmations I am...

Evening

Time:_____

Three amazing things that happened today...

How could I have made today better?

Morning

Time:_____ Date: / /

I am grateful for...

- An old relationship:

- An opportunity you have today:

- Something good/great that happened yesterday:

- Something small:

Daily affirmations I am...

Evening

Time:_____

Three amazing things that happened today...

How could I have made today better?

Morning

I am grateful for...

- An old relationship:

- An opportunity you have today:

- Something good/great that happened yesterday:

- Something small:

Daily affirmations I am...

Evening

Time:_____

Three amazing things that happened today...

How could I have made today better?

Morning

Time:_____ Date: / /

I am grateful for...

- An old relationship:

- An opportunity you have today:

- Something good/great that happened yesterday:

- Something small:

Daily affirmations I am...

Evening

Time:_____

Three amazing things that happened today...

How could I have made today better?

Morning

Time:_____ Date: / /

I am grateful for...

- An old relationship:

- An opportunity you have today:

- Something good/great that happened yesterday:

- Something small:

Daily affirmations I am...

Evening

Time:_____

Three amazing things that happened today...

How could I have made today better?

Morning

Time:_____ Date: / /

I am grateful for...

- An old relationship:

- An opportunity you have today:

- Something good/great that happened yesterday:

- Something small:

Daily affirmations I am...

Evening

Time:_____

Three amazing things that happened today...

How could I have made today better?

Morning

I am grateful for...

- An old relationship:

- An opportunity you have today:

- Something good/great that happened yesterday:

- Something small:

Daily affirmations I am...

Evening

Time:_____

Three amazing things that happened today...

How could I have made today better?

Morning

Time:_____ Date: / /

I am grateful for...

- An old relationship:

- An opportunity you have today:

- Something good/great that happened yesterday:

- Something small:

Daily affirmations I am...

Evening

Time:_____

Three amazing things that happened today...

How could I have made today better?

Morning

I am grateful for...

- An old relationship:

- An opportunity you have today:

- Something good/great that happened yesterday:

- Something small:

Daily affirmations I am...

Evening

Time:_____

Three amazing things that happened today...

How could I have made today better?

Morning

I am grateful for...

- • An old relationship:

- • An opportunity you have today:

- • Something good/great that happened yesterday:

- • Something small:

Daily affirmations I am...

Evening

Time:_____

Three amazing things that happened today...

How could I have made today better?

Morning

Time:_____ Date: / /

I am grateful for...

- An old relationship:

- An opportunity you have today:

- Something good/great that happened yesterday:

- Something small:

Daily affirmations I am...

Evening

Time:_____

Three amazing things that happened today...

How could I have made today better?

Morning   Time:_____ Date: / /

I am grateful for...

- An old relationship:

- An opportunity you have today:

- Something good/great that happened yesterday:

- Something small:

Daily affirmations I am...

Evening   Time:_____

Three amazing things that happened today...

How could I have made today better?

Morning

Time:_____ Date: / /

I am grateful for...

- An old relationship:

- An opportunity you have today:

- Something good/great that happened yesterday:

- Something small:

Daily affirmations I am...

Evening

Time:_____

Three amazing things that happened today...

How could I have made today better?

Morning

I am grateful for...

- An old relationship:

- An opportunity you have today:

- Something good/great that happened yesterday:

- Something small:

Daily affirmations I am...

Evening

Time:_____

Three amazing things that happened today...

How could I have made today better?

Morning

I am grateful for...

- An old relationship:

- An opportunity you have today:

- Something good/great that happened yesterday:

- Something small:

Daily affirmations I am...

Evening

Time:_____

Three amazing things that happened today...

How could I have made today better?

Morning

Time:_____ Date: / /

I am grateful for...

- An old relationship:

- An opportunity you have today:

- Something good/great that happened yesterday:

- Something small:

Daily affirmations I am...

Evening

Time:_____

Three amazing things that happened today...

How could I have made today better?

Morning

I am grateful for...

- An old relationship:

- An opportunity you have today:

- Something good/great that happened yesterday:

- Something small:

Daily affirmations I am...

Evening

Time:_____

Three amazing things that happened today...

How could I have made today better?

Morning

I am grateful for...

- An old relationship:

- An opportunity you have today:

- Something good/great that happened yesterday:

- Something small:

Daily affirmations I am...

Evening

Time:_____

Three amazing things that happened today...

How could I have made today better?

Morning

Time:_____ Date: / /

I am grateful for...

- An old relationship:

- An opportunity you have today:

- Something good/great that happened yesterday:

- Something small:

Daily affirmations I am...

Evening

Time:_____

Three amazing things that happened today...

How could I have made today better?

Morning   Time:_____ Date: / /

I am grateful for...

- • An old relationship:

- • An opportunity you have today:

- • Something good/great that happened yesterday:

- • Something small:

Daily affirmations I am...

Evening   Time:_____

Three amazing things that happened today...

How could I have made today better?

Morning

Time:_____ Date: / /

I am grateful for...

- An old relationship:

- An opportunity you have today:

- Something good/great that happened yesterday:

- Something small:

Daily affirmations I am...

Evening

Time:_____

Three amazing things that happened today...

How could I have made today better?

Morning

Time:_____ Date: / /

I am grateful for...

- An old relationship:

- An opportunity you have today:

- Something good/great that happened yesterday:

- Something small:

Daily affirmations I am...

Evening

Time:_____

Three amazing things that happened today...

How could I have made today better?

Morning

I am grateful for...

- An old relationship:

- An opportunity you have today:

- Something good/great that happened yesterday:

- Something small:

Daily affirmations I am...

Evening

Time:_____

Three amazing things that happened today...

How could I have made today better?

Morning

Time:_____ Date: / /

I am grateful for...

- An old relationship:

- An opportunity you have today:

- Something good/great that happened yesterday:

- Something small:

Daily affirmations I am...

Evening

Time:_____

Three amazing things that happened today...

How could I have made today better?

Morning

Time:_____ Date: / /

I am grateful for...

- An old relationship:

- An opportunity you have today:

- Something good/great that happened yesterday:

- Something small:

Daily affirmations I am...

Evening

Time:_____

Three amazing things that happened today...

How could I have made today better?

Morning

Time:_____ Date: / /

I am grateful for...

- An old relationship:

- An opportunity you have today:

- Something good/great that happened yesterday:

- Something small:

Daily affirmations I am...

Evening

Time:_____

Three amazing things that happened today...

How could I have made today better?

Morning

I am grateful for...

- An old relationship:

- An opportunity you have today:

- Something good/great that happened yesterday:

- Something small:

Daily affirmations I am...

Evening

Time:_____

Three amazing things that happened today...

How could I have made today better?

Morning   Time:_____ Date: / /

I am grateful for...

- • An old relationship:

- • An opportunity you have today:

- • Something good/great that happened yesterday:

- • Something small:

Daily affirmations I am...

Evening   Time:_____

Three amazing things that happened today...

How could I have made today better?

Morning

Time:_____ Date: / /

I am grateful for...

- An old relationship:

- An opportunity you have today:

- Something good/great that happened yesterday:

- Something small:

Daily affirmations I am...

Evening

Time:_____

Three amazing things that happened today...

How could I have made today better?

Morning

I am grateful for...

- An old relationship:

- An opportunity you have today:

- Something good/great that happened yesterday:

- Something small:

Daily affirmations I am...

Evening

Time:_____

Three amazing things that happened today...

How could I have made today better?

Morning

I am grateful for...

- An old relationship:

- An opportunity you have today:

- Something good/great that happened yesterday:

- Something small:

Daily affirmations I am...

Evening

Time:_____

Three amazing things that happened today...

How could I have made today better?

Morning   Time:_____ Date: / /

I am grateful for...

- • An old relationship:

- • An opportunity you have today:

- • Something good/great that happened yesterday:

- • Something small:

Daily affirmations I am...

Evening   Time:_____

Three amazing things that happened today...

How could I have made today better?

Morning

I am grateful for...

- An old relationship:

- An opportunity you have today:

- Something good/great that happened yesterday:

- Something small:

Daily affirmations I am...

Evening

Time:_____

Three amazing things that happened today...

How could I have made today better?

Morning

Time:_____   Date: / /

I am grateful for...

- An old relationship:

- An opportunity you have today:

- Something good/great that happened yesterday:

- Something small:

Daily affirmations I am...

Evening

Time:_____

Three amazing things that happened today...

How could I have made today better?

247

Morning

I am grateful for...

- An old relationship:

- An opportunity you have today:

- Something good/great that happened yesterday:

- Something small:

Daily affirmations I am...

Evening

Time:_____

Three amazing things that happened today...

How could I have made today better?

Morning

Time:_____ Date: / /

I am grateful for...

- An old relationship:

- An opportunity you have today:

- Something good/great that happened yesterday:

- Something small:

Daily affirmations I am...

Evening

Time:_____

Three amazing things that happened today...

How could I have made today better?

Morning

I am grateful for...

- An old relationship:

- An opportunity you have today:

- Something good/great that happened yesterday:

- Something small:

Daily affirmations I am...

Evening

Time:_____

Three amazing things that happened today...

How could I have made today better?

Morning   Time:_____ Date: / /

I am grateful for...

- An old relationship:

- An opportunity you have today:

- Something good/great that happened yesterday:

- Something small:

Daily affirmations I am...

Evening   Time:_____

Three amazing things that happened today...

How could I have made today better?

Morning

Time:_____ Date: / /

I am grateful for...

- An old relationship:

- An opportunity you have today:

- Something good/great that happened yesterday:

- Something small:

Daily affirmations I am...

Evening

Time:_____

Three amazing things that happened today...

How could I have made today better?

Morning

Time:_____ Date: / /

I am grateful for...

- An old relationship:

- An opportunity you have today:

- Something good/great that happened yesterday:

- Something small:

Daily affirmations I am...

Evening

Time:_____

Three amazing things that happened today...

How could I have made today better?

Morning

Time:_____ Date: / /

I am grateful for...

- An old relationship:

- An opportunity you have today:

- Something good/great that happened yesterday:

- Something small:

Daily affirmations I am...

Evening

Time:_____

Three amazing things that happened today...

How could I have made today better?

Morning

Time:_____ Date: / /

I am grateful for...

- An old relationship:

- An opportunity you have today:

- Something good/great that happened yesterday:

- Something small:

Daily affirmations I am...

Evening

Time:_____

Three amazing things that happened today...

How could I have made today better?

Morning

I am grateful for...

- An old relationship:

- An opportunity you have today:

- Something good/great that happened yesterday:

- Something small:

Daily affirmations I am...

Evening

Time:_____

Three amazing things that happened today...

How could I have made today better?

Morning

Time:_____ Date: / /

I am grateful for...

- An old relationship:

- An opportunity you have today:

- Something good/great that happened yesterday:

- Something small:

Daily affirmations I am...

Evening

Time:_____

Three amazing things that happened today...

How could I have made today better?

Morning

Time:_____ Date: / /

I am grateful for...

- An old relationship:

- An opportunity you have today:

- Something good/great that happened yesterday:

- Something small:

Daily affirmations I am...

Evening

Time:_____

Three amazing things that happened today...

How could I have made today better?

Morning

I am grateful for...

- An old relationship:

- An opportunity you have today:

- Something good/great that happened yesterday:

- Something small:

Daily affirmations I am...

Evening

Time:_____

Three amazing things that happened today...

How could I have made today better?

Morning

Time:_____ Date: / /

I am grateful for...

- An old relationship:

- An opportunity you have today:

- Something good/great that happened yesterday:

- Something small:

Daily affirmations I am...

Evening

Time:_____

Three amazing things that happened today...

How could I have made today better?

Morning   Time:_____ Date: / /

I am grateful for...

- An old relationship:

- An opportunity you have today:

- Something good/great that happened yesterday:

- Something small:

Daily affirmations I am...

Evening   Time:_____

Three amazing things that happened today...

How could I have made today better?

Morning

I am grateful for...

- An old relationship:

- An opportunity you have today:

- Something good/great that happened yesterday:

- Something small:

Daily affirmations I am...

Evening

Time:_____

Three amazing things that happened today...

How could I have made today better?

Morning

I am grateful for...

- An old relationship:

- An opportunity you have today:

- Something good/great that happened yesterday:

- Something small:

Daily affirmations I am...

Evening

Time:_____

Three amazing things that happened today...

How could I have made today better?

Morning

Time:_____ Date: / /

I am grateful for...

- An old relationship:

- An opportunity you have today:

- Something good/great that happened yesterday:

- Something small:

Daily affirmations I am...

Evening

Time:_____

Three amazing things that happened today...

How could I have made today better?

Morning

I am grateful for...

- An old relationship:

- An opportunity you have today:

- Something good/great that happened yesterday:

- Something small:

Daily affirmations I am...

Evening

Three amazing things that happened today...

How could I have made today better?

Morning

Time:_____ Date: / /

I am grateful for...

- An old relationship:

- An opportunity you have today:

- Something good/great that happened yesterday:

- Something small:

Daily affirmations I am...

Evening

Time:_____

Three amazing things that happened today...

How could I have made today better?

Morning

I am grateful for...

- An old relationship:

- An opportunity you have today:

- Something good/great that happened yesterday:

- Something small:

Daily affirmations I am...

Evening

Time:_____

Three amazing things that happened today...

How could I have made today better?

Morning

I am grateful for...

- An old relationship:

- An opportunity you have today:

- Something good/great that happened yesterday:

- Something small:

Daily affirmations I am...

Evening

Time:_____

Three amazing things that happened today...

How could I have made today better?

Morning \qquad Time:_____ Date: / /

I am grateful for...

- An old relationship:

- An opportunity you have today:

- Something good/great that happened yesterday:

- Something small:

Daily affirmations I am...

Evening \qquad Time:_____

Three amazing things that happened today...

How could I have made today better?

Morning

I am grateful for...

- An old relationship:

- An opportunity you have today:

- Something good/great that happened yesterday:

- Something small:

Daily affirmations I am...

Evening

Time:_____

Three amazing things that happened today...

How could I have made today better?

Morning

Time:_____ Date: / /

I am grateful for...

- An old relationship:

- An opportunity you have today:

- Something good/great that happened yesterday:

- Something small:

Daily affirmations I am...

Evening

Time:_____

Three amazing things that happened today...

How could I have made today better?

Morning

Time:_____ Date: / /

I am grateful for...

- An old relationship:

- An opportunity you have today:

- Something good/great that happened yesterday:

- Something small:

Daily affirmations I am...

Evening

Time:_____

Three amazing things that happened today...

How could I have made today better?

Morning   Time:_____ Date: / /

I am grateful for...

- • An old relationship:

- • An opportunity you have today:

- • Something good/great that happened yesterday:

- • Something small:

Daily affirmations I am...

Evening   Time:_____

Three amazing things that happened today...

How could I have made today better?

Morning

I am grateful for...

- An old relationship:

- An opportunity you have today:

- Something good/great that happened yesterday:

- Something small:

Daily affirmations I am...

Evening

Time:_____

Three amazing things that happened today...

How could I have made today better?

Morning

I am grateful for...

- An old relationship:

- An opportunity you have today:

- Something good/great that happened yesterday:

- Something small:

Daily affirmations I am...

Evening

Time:_____

Three amazing things that happened today...

How could I have made today better?

Morning

I am grateful for...

- An old relationship:

- An opportunity you have today:

- Something good/great that happened yesterday:

- Something small:

Daily affirmations I am...

Evening

Time:_____

Three amazing things that happened today...

How could I have made today better?

Morning

Time:_____   Date: / /

I am grateful for...

- An old relationship:

- An opportunity you have today:

- Something good/great that happened yesterday:

- Something small:

Daily affirmations I am...

Evening

Time:_____

Three amazing things that happened today...

How could I have made today better?

Morning

I am grateful for...

- An old relationship:

- An opportunity you have today:

- Something good/great that happened yesterday:

- Something small:

Daily affirmations I am...

Evening

Time:_____

Three amazing things that happened today...

How could I have made today better?

Morning

I am grateful for...

- An old relationship:

- An opportunity you have today:

- Something good/great that happened yesterday:

- Something small:

Daily affirmations I am...

Evening

Time:_____

Three amazing things that happened today...

How could I have made today better?

Morning

Time:_____ Date: / /

I am grateful for...

- An old relationship:

- An opportunity you have today:

- Something good/great that happened yesterday:

- Something small:

Daily affirmations I am...

Evening

Time:_____

Three amazing things that happened today...

How could I have made today better?

Morning   Time:_____ Date: / /

I am grateful for...

- An old relationship:

- An opportunity you have today:

- Something good/great that happened yesterday:

- Something small:

Daily affirmations I am...

Evening   Time:_____

Three amazing things that happened today...

How could I have made today better?

Morning

Time:_____ Date: / /

I am grateful for...

- An old relationship:

- An opportunity you have today:

- Something good/great that happened yesterday:

- Something small:

Daily affirmations I am...

Evening

Time:_____

Three amazing things that happened today...

How could I have made today better?

Morning   Time:_____ Date: / /

I am grateful for...

- An old relationship:

- An opportunity you have today:

- Something good/great that happened yesterday:

- Something small:

Daily affirmations I am...

Evening   Time:_____

Three amazing things that happened today...

How could I have made today better?

Morning

Time:_____ Date: / /

I am grateful for...

- An old relationship:

- An opportunity you have today:

- Something good/great that happened yesterday:

- Something small:

Daily affirmations I am...

Evening

Time:_____

Three amazing things that happened today...

How could I have made today better?

Morning   Time:_____ Date: / /

I am grateful for...

- •   An old relationship:

- •   An opportunity you have today:

- •   Something good/great that happened yesterday:

- •   Something small:

Daily affirmations I am...

Evening   Time:_____

Three amazing things that happened today...

How could I have made today better?

Morning

Time:_____ Date: / /

I am grateful for...

- An old relationship:

- An opportunity you have today:

- Something good/great that happened yesterday:

- Something small:

Daily affirmations I am...

Evening

Time:_____

Three amazing things that happened today...

How could I have made today better?

Morning   Time:_____   Date: / /

I am grateful for...

- An old relationship:

- An opportunity you have today:

- Something good/great that happened yesterday:

- Something small:

Daily affirmations I am...

Evening   Time:_____

Three amazing things that happened today...

How could I have made today better?

Morning

Time:_____ Date: / /

I am grateful for...

- An old relationship:

- An opportunity you have today:

- Something good/great that happened yesterday:

- Something small:

Daily affirmations I am...

Evening

Time:_____

Three amazing things that happened today...

How could I have made today better?

Morning

Time:_____   Date: / /

I am grateful for...

- An old relationship:

- An opportunity you have today:

- Something good/great that happened yesterday:

- Something small:

Daily affirmations I am...

Evening

Time:_____

Three amazing things that happened today...

How could I have made today better?

Morning

I am grateful for...

- An old relationship:

- An opportunity you have today:

- Something good/great that happened yesterday:

- Something small:

Daily affirmations I am...

Evening

Time:_____

Three amazing things that happened today...

How could I have made today better?

Morning   Time:_____ Date: / /

I am grateful for...

- An old relationship:

- An opportunity you have today:

- Something good/great that happened yesterday:

- Something small:

Daily affirmations I am...

Evening   Time:_____

Three amazing things that happened today...

How could I have made today better?

Morning

Time:_____ Date: / /

I am grateful for...

- An old relationship:

- An opportunity you have today:

- Something good/great that happened yesterday:

- Something small:

Daily affirmations I am...

Evening

Time:_____

Three amazing things that happened today...

How could I have made today better?

Morning
Time:_____   Date: / /

I am grateful for...

- An old relationship:

- An opportunity you have today:

- Something good/great that happened yesterday:

- Something small:

Daily affirmations I am...

Evening
Time:_____

Three amazing things that happened today...

How could I have made today better?

Morning

I am grateful for...

- An old relationship:

- An opportunity you have today:

- Something good/great that happened yesterday:

- Something small:

Daily affirmations I am...

Evening

Time:_____

Three amazing things that happened today...

How could I have made today better?

Morning   Time:_____   Date: / /

I am grateful for...

- An old relationship:

- An opportunity you have today:

- Something good/great that happened yesterday:

- Something small:

Daily affirmations I am...

Evening   Time:_____

Three amazing things that happened today...

How could I have made today better?

Morning

I am grateful for...

- An old relationship:

- An opportunity you have today:

- Something good/great that happened yesterday:

- Something small:

Daily affirmations I am...

Evening

Time:_____

Three amazing things that happened today...

How could I have made today better?

Morning

I am grateful for...

- An old relationship:

- An opportunity you have today:

- Something good/great that happened yesterday:

- Something small:

Daily affirmations I am...

Evening

Time:_____

Three amazing things that happened today...

How could I have made today better?

Morning

I am grateful for...

- An old relationship:

- An opportunity you have today:

- Something good/great that happened yesterday:

- Something small:

Daily affirmations I am...

Evening

Time:_____

Three amazing things that happened today...

How could I have made today better?

Morning

I am grateful for...

- An old relationship:

- An opportunity you have today:

- Something good/great that happened yesterday:

- Something small:

Daily affirmations I am...

Evening

Time:_____

Three amazing things that happened today...

How could I have made today better?

Morning

I am grateful for...

- An old relationship:

- An opportunity you have today:

- Something good/great that happened yesterday:

- Something small:

Daily affirmations I am...

Evening

Time:_____

Three amazing things that happened today...

How could I have made today better?

Made in the USA
Middletown, DE
17 May 2017